I0479804

9 POWERFUL METHODS TO STOP STRESS.

Practicing this techniques will definitely give you an hedge over stress.

By

Dr DOUGLAS JASON

Copyright © (DR DOUGLAS JASON) 2023. All rights reserved

Before this document is duplicated or reproduced in any manner, the publisher's consent must be gained.

Therefore, the contents within can neither be stored electronically, transferred, nor kept in a database. Neither in part nor in full can the document be copied, scanned, faxed, or retained without approval from the publisher or creator.

TABLE OF CONTENT

ABOUT THE AUTHOR

INTRODUCTION

TABLE OF CONTENTS

9 POWERFUL METHODS TO STOP STRESS.

Practicing this techniques will definitely give you an hedge over stress.

INTRODUCTION

CHAPTER 1
Break out the bubble gum

CHAPTER 2
Go outside.

CHAPTER 3:
Smile Sincerely.

CHAPTER 4
Sniff Some Lavender

CHAPTER 5
Listen Up.

CHAPTER 6
REBOOT YOUR BREATH

CHAPTER 7
Be kind to yourself

CHAPTER 8

Write Your Stress Away

CHAPTER 9
Tell a Friend,

CONCLUSIONS

Dr. Douglas Jason is a certified dietician who has a strong passion for wellness and a big eagerness to help people all over the world. He uses healthy food, herbs, spices, and other useful tools to help mankind realize its overall goal of optimum health.

INTRODUCTION

Place the stress it deserves Life will always involve some level of stress. Your physical and emotional states are affected by how you handle them. Here are 9 relaxing techniques you can apply right away to reduce tension and enter a more relaxed state. The next time you're looking for a technique to reduce stress, try one of these tactics.

CHAPTER 1

Break out the bubble gum

Feeling a little disjointed right now? Pick up a piece of gum. According to research, chewing gum can help reduce tension and anxiety. It's possible that chewing rhythmically increases blood flow to the brain. According to a different viewpoint, the flavor and aroma of the gum trigger the relaxation response. Grab a stick of gum the next time you feel like you can't stop worrying; it works well, is cheap, and is something you can do almost anywhere.

CHAPTER 2

Go outside.

Do you want to learn how to quit worrying? Step outdoors. Going outside is a fantastic stress reliever. According to studies, going outside for a short while, even close to home can improve your mood. Natural environments not only promote relaxation but are outside frequently including physical activity as well.

CHAPTER 3:

Smile Sincerely.

Don't worry, just grin! The saying "Grin and bear it" has some truth to it. When you smile, your facial muscles become slightly tense, which helps to relieve stress. Genuine smiles that engage the muscles surrounding the mouth and eyes are particularly effective at reducing stress. When a stressful scenario has gone, smiling might also help a raised heart rate recover more quickly.

CHAPTER 4

Sniff Some Lavender

Looking for a way to reduce stress at work? Grab the lavender. Some scents can induce tranquility. In one study, the stress levels of nurses with and without lavender oil vials pinned to their clothing were examined. Compared to the nurses who were scent-free, those who were exposed to the lavender scent said they felt more at ease. The effects of painkillers and anti-anxiety medications can be enhanced by lavender. If you use one of these medications, make sure to consult a doctor before taking lavender oil. Additionally, migraines and tension headaches may benefit from the use of lavender essential oil.

CHAPTER 5

Listen Up.

Music might help you stay calm whether you have to give a presentation at work or are dealing with another stressful situation. One study found that listening to Latin choral music, namely Miserere by Gregorio Allegri, reduced cortisol levels in participants more than listening to the sound of rippling water alone. Unwinding by listening to calming music is among the

simplest ways to reduce
stress.

CHAPTER 6

REBOOT YOUR BREATH

One method to swiftly cease the stress response is to do breathing exercises. Exercises that include breathing have two relaxing effects. By concentrating on the breath, one can divert focus from anxious and scary thoughts as well as halt the body's "fight or flight" reaction. To carry out the exercise, inhale slowly and deeply through your nose. Allow the air to fill your abdomen and chest to expand. Repeating a word or phrase that calms and soothes you as you exhale should take up the same amount of time as your inhalation. The best results come from breathing exercises that you do for at least 10 minutes.

CHAPTER 7

Be kind to yourself

Every person has an internal dialogue going on. Sometimes we don't use gentle, soothing language while talking to ourselves. You can stay calm and find answers to issues more easily if you learn the skill of compassionate and empowering self-talk. When faced with a challenge or distressing circumstance, consider how you would approach a buddy who was going through a comparable predicament. It's much more reassuring to tell yourself, "I can figure this out," or "It'll be OK," rather than to catastrophize or use negative self-talk. Try talking to yourself the way you would to a distressed friend in need the next time you wonder how to stop being so stressed.

CHAPTER 8

Write Your Stress Away

Do you feel stressed? You may feel more at ease and come up with new answers to your problems as a result of journaling your issues. These advantages can be attained by writing in a journal, a computer file, or even a phone app. The best results come from being open and honest about your emotions.

When you're uncertain, consult your journal.

How to reduce school anxiety
What can I do to stop stress eating?
How to lessen your stress
How to prevent weight gain due to stress
How to stop stress-related sobbing
How to relax and quit worrying about everything

You can manage your stress and anxiety by keeping a journal.

CHAPTER 9

Tell a Friend,

A major source of stress relief is social support. When you're feeling pressured, get together with friends or family members. Find someone to hang out with who is facing comparable difficulties. You will feel less alone if you talk about your experiences with people who can relate.

CONCLUSIONS

Many factors affect mood during exercise. Engaging in physical activity can help you forget about daily concerns. It also releases endorphins, which improve mood. Any form of exercise, whether you like long walks or working out in the gym, lowers ten tension and anxiety.

www.ingramcontent.com/pod-product-compliance
Lightning Source LLC
Chambersburg PA
CBHW071126220526

45467CB00004B/2076